STOP NEGATIVE
THINKING

HOW TO STOP WORRYING,
RELIEVE STRESS, AND BECOME
A HAPPY PERSON AGAIN

Doc Orman, M.D.

Cambria font used with permission from Microsoft.

Published By:

TRO Productions, LLC
P.O. Box 768
Sparks, Maryland 21152

In association with TCK Publishing

www.TCKPublishing.com

DISCLAIMERS AND LEGAL NOTICES

Both the author and publisher of this book have strived to be as accurate and complete as possible in the creation of this information product. While all attempts have been made to verify the accuracy of the information contained herein, there is no warranty either expressly stated or implied of complete or permanent accuracy. After all, knowledge does evolve and change.

The author and publisher and any subsequent distributors of this work also assume no responsibility for any errors, assumptions, or interpretations you might make as result of consuming this information. You are solely responsible for how you choose to understand and make use of this information. Please use prudent judgment in attempting to apply any strategies, exercises, or other recommendations suggested herein. Also, any perceived slights of specific persons, peoples, or organizations are unintentional.

This book is also not intended to be a substitute or replacement for competent medical or psychological treatment when these may be needed. If you suffer from very severe anxiety, severe phobias, severe depression or any other serious mental health condition, the advice in this book may not be appropriate or sufficient for you. You are advised to consult and work with an experienced mental health professional, if you are not already doing so.

Also, if you believe that your symptoms or your problems are beginning to get worse as you read this book, you should stop reading it immediately and consult a trained health professional.

Dr. Mort Orman is a board-certified Internal Medicine physician. While he has been successfully helping and coaching people to overcome their stress and anxiety related problems for more than 30 years, he is not a licensed or practicing mental health professional. Therefore, you need to evaluate and personally assess all advice and suggestions put forth in this book in this light.

Bottom line: you are 100% responsible for how you interpret and make use of the information in this book. So please do so wisely.

CONTENTS

WHY YOU SHOULD
READ THIS BOOK

There's no question about it - being a negative thinker can cause lots of problems, conflicts, and other types of stress in your life. Here are just a few examples:

> *You can poison your relationships with others by being overly negative, critical, and judgmental.*

> *You frequently become angry because you think everyone around you is always doing things 'wrong'.*

> *You fail to take advantage of great opportunities that come your way by focusing too much on risks and not enough on possibilities.*

> *You may become depressed and despondent if you constantly view life through a negative filter.*

NEGATIVE THINKING IS VERY PERVASIVE ... AND VERY SEDUCTIVE

Negative thinking is so pervasive in our society today that it is frequently mistaken for healthy, realistic thinking. Yes, negative things can and do happen. But a large part of our negative thinking is not truly justified. It's simply automatic thinking that has little correspondence to either truth or reality.

Negative thinking has become so pervasive and automatic for a number of reasons. One reason is that growing up as young children, we often get lots of critical input from our parents and other caretakers, who (with good intentions) tend to point out the many flaws in our behaviors. Another reason is that the news media and entertainment industries tend to focus more on negative themes than on positive ones, simply because tragedies, disasters, crime, violence, and other negative occurrences seem to grab our attention, and heighten our emotions, much more powerfully than positive stories or images of positive events.

There are probably many other reasons as well. The bottom line, however, is that negative thinking is very seductive...and most of us tend to automatically engage in it way more than we should.

Negative Thinking And Emotions

All of our negative emotions have their roots in negative thinking. You can't get angry without engaging in negative thinking. You can't feel worried or afraid without being concerned that something bad or harmful is likely to happen to you or to someone you care about. And you can't feel frustrated, guilty, sad, or depressed without very specific negative thinking driving your feelings at a very deep level.

WHY I WROTE THIS BOOK

Hi. My name is Mort (Doc) Orman, M.D. and I am a physician, author, stress coach and founder of The Stress Mastery Academy.

I'd like to welcome you to this self-help success guide about how you can stop being such a negative thinker.

If you've been struggling to stop, change or control your negative thinking, without much success, this guide may finally show you how to achieve the relief you've been hoping and searching for.

This success guide will not only show you why your efforts so far have gone unrewarded, but it will also introduce you to some new and different approaches to finally win your battle against your own negative thinking.

In this guide, you're going to learn why most of the advice for reducing negative thinking that's being offered to people today doesn't work. You're going to learn why positive thinking doesn't work, why repeating positive affirmations over and over again doesn't work, and even why trying to stop your negative thoughts from occurring doesn't work either.

None of these commonly offered strategies are powerful enough to get you where you want to go. And while they might look good in theory, they are no match at all for the strength and the depth of all the negative thoughts within you.

There are strategies that can work, however, and I'm going to share some of them with you here.

Your Blueprint For Success

This guide will give you a ten-point blueprint to follow for eliminating most of the adverse effects negative thinking may be producing in your life. If you study this blueprint carefully, and apply the simple recommendations I'm going to offer you here, you should be well on your way to becoming a more positive, optimistic person.

Here is a quick glimpse of what each of the ten points in your success plan will cover:

1. Why negative thinking isn't the problem...something else is!

2. Why the more focused you are, the less intelligent you appear.

3. The number one thinking habit that repeatedly gets you into trouble (either you think this way or you don't).

4. Why you can't stop thinking negatively even if you want to (even if you really, really, really want to).

5. There are a lot of things in the 'box' called 'life'...except for this.

6. If you think tax assessments are bad...this one's even worse.

7. Do you know what your current relationship to negative thinking is (and why you should change it)?

8. What is the best relationship to have towards negative thinking?

9. How often do you suppose you are wrong? (now multiply that by 10)

10. What is 'flipping to the opposite reality' and how can it help you to finally see the light?

WHY THE QUICK FIX MENTALITY IS BROKEN

I am very confident that if you follow the ten point plan contained in this guide, you will be able to conquer your negative thinking   successfully. However, you must be clear from the start that this plan is not a quick-fix approach.

If you are serious about wanting to overcome your negative thinking problem, you are going to have to work at it. I'm sure you already know that. But sometimes when people hear lofty promises, like the ones I just made, they think some magical quick-fix solution is about to be delivered to them.

Well, there's nothing magical about the ten point plan you're going to get here. Don't get me wrong...it's a really good plan...probably the best strategic and tactical blueprint for dealing with negative thinking you will find anywhere.

But it's not a quick-fix, and it definitely won't do anything beneficial for you, if all you do is read about it. It's a plan that needs to be 'worked' if you're going to get any lasting results. First, it needs to be fully understood (that's the reading part). Then, it needs to be put into action (this is your part).

The only way to change or overcome any habit of thinking is to have a good game plan for doing so, and then practice deploying that game plan as many times as you need to in order to achieve your desired goals.

I can give you the game plan and show you why it makes sense. But only you can apply this plan, and tailor it to your own unique life circumstances. So, now that my little motivational pep talk is out of the way, let's get down to serious business.

1

NEGATIVE THINKING ISN'T YOUR PROBLEM... SOMETHING ELSE IS!

I bet you assumed, from the title of this guide, that helping you stop your negative thinking is the aim of this guide. Well, it's not!

There are two very good reasons why it's not...and why you should be happy that it's not.

First, I'm going to show you in this guide that if you are now a frequent negative thinker, you're not going to be able to stop thinking negatively. At least not in the short run.

The second, more important reason, is that negative thinking isn't your real problem anyway. Something else is.

That 'something else' is that you actually believe most of your negative thoughts. It's believing your negative thoughts are true that is the crux of your problem. And unless you attack this deeper 'believing problem' directly and much more powerfully than you've done up to now, you don't really stand a chance of removing all the damage that negative thinking can do in your life.

In addition, once you learn how to handle your 'believing problem', you won't even need to stop, change, or control your negative thinking anymore. In addition to knowing that this is not even a realistic goal, you'll discover that your repeated negative thoughts can actually become quite useful to you. Instead of hoping and dreaming about finally getting rid of them, you may just find yourself enjoying them and appreciating them for the value they can bring to you...if approached in some of the ways I'm going to share with you later in this guide.

NOTE: It's important to point out that negative thinking is not always a bad thing. Many famous, successful, and very accomplished people are inveterate negative thinkers. In addition, being successful in many types of jobs and professions requires a healthy dose of appropriate negative thinking.

For example, you can't be a good lawyer and not rely upon negative thinking abilities. You can't be a good detective or police officer without engaging in negative thinking frequently. The problem with negative thinking is when it leads to unwanted problems and outcomes in your life. This is the aspect of negative thinking that most people do want to learn how to overcome, and this is what this guide is designed to help you do.

2

WHAT DOES FOCUS HAVE TO DO WITH NEGATIVE THINKING?

Before we get into specifics about how to best deal with your negative thinking, you need to better understand how and why you became such a negative thinker.

It's really no surprise that you and millions of other people alive today are extremely negative thinkers. Our Western culture tends to foster negative thinking, for reasons I mentioned earlier.

There are two major aspects of negative thinking, however, which are very important for you to understand. They can be summed up by the terms focus and automaticity. Let me explain.

FOCUS RESULTS IN 'BLINDNESS'

Negative thinking usually involves a very limited, narrow focus of your attention.

Focusing exclusively on just the negative side of any occurrence in our lives makes us more or less blind to any opposite (i.e. positive) perspectives.

Thus, when we believe someone is out to get us, or otherwise do us harm, it's often hard for us to consider, at the very same time, that we may be wrong about our assumption, or that the other person may actually have good intentions at heart.

Of course, sometimes people really are out to get us. And when this happens, an appropriate dose of realistic negative thinking can be very beneficial. But more often than we like to admit, our automatic negative assumptions are not entirely accurate.

This brings us to the second key understanding - automaticity.

MUCH OF OUR NEGATIVE THINKING IS AUTOMATIC AND CONDITIONED

As we go through life, negative thoughts, beliefs, opinions, perceptions, emotions, etc., routinely get triggered within us. For some people, this can happen hundreds of times every day.

Some of these negative thoughts, feelings etc., will be appropriate - in other words, they will be more or less consistent with reality. But many will not.

Such is the nature of being human. We all have bodies that get conditioned, throughout our lives, to react automatically to a wide range of triggering events.

If you are a negative thinker now, all this means is that you (i.e. your body) has been conditioned to automatically react by focusing on negatives (rather than positives, or equally balanced views). For many of us, this conditioning dates back to the time we were small children.

A PERFECT STORM

When you put the following facts together, you'll see that they lead to a type of 'perfect storm' that has caused us to become so negative in our ways of looking at life:

- ➤ *Many of us have been conditioned over many years to automatically focus on negatives, rather than on more positive perspectives;*

- ➤ *Our automatic, conditioned ways of thinking are often way too narrow in their scope, and this renders us blind to other actual, legitimate aspects of reality;*

> ➢ *Our automatic, conditioned ways of thinking are often inconsistent with the truth about life or about whatever may have really happened.*

Hopefully, you can see now how automatic negative thinking, limited focus (and partial blindness), and failing to appreciate the full truth about whatever happens in life all combine with each other to produce many potential problems and stress in our lives.

The good news is that much of this stress can either be prevented or eliminated, once you know how to successfully deal with your conditioned negative thinking tendencies.

3

THE KILLER
THINKING HABIT

Just to give you one example of how focus and automatic thinking can lead to problems and stress in your life, let's take a closer look at one very common thinking pattern that frequently gets us into trouble.

This pattern of thinking is called Either/Or Thinking. It's very common to acquire this habit of thinking as you grow up in our society…and in most other Western societies as well.

WHAT IS EITHER/OR THINKING?

Either/Or Thinking is our tendency to automatically view the world around us, and many of the events that happen within it, from an either/or framework.

With Either/Or Thinking, we tend to view life as occurring in very discrete, polarized opposites. Something happens, and we view it as being either good or bad. Someone does something or says something, and we view it as being either right or being wrong. Something goes well, and we look for people to credit. Something goes poorly, and we look for people to blame.

In other words, we tend to view many aspects of life from highly polarized Either/Or dichotomies. Something can be either black, or it can be white. But if it is black, it can't be white, and so on.

THE PROBLEM WITH EITHER/OR THINKING

While Either/Or Thinking may seem like a convenient way of simplifying our life, it can lead to faulty impressions and assumptions that can cause us to experience stress. The reason is that life rarely happens in nice, neat, exclusively one-sided ways.

Life is usually much more complex and multidimensional. So when we focus exclusively on just one side of a complex dualistic reality, it appears to be one-sided, when in truth it is not.

For example, life rarely happens in exclusively good or exclusively bad ways.

Most things that happen have both good and bad qualities at the same time. Or they can have potentially good and bad future possibilities to them. Eastern cultures have embraced this dualistic nature of reality with their 'Yin-Yang' way of thinking, where aspects of life are viewed as always having a broader spectrum of qualities, including both sides of a dichotomy, even though they may appear to have only one.

This pattern of Either/Or Thinking is particularly active in negative thinkers, who automatically tend to get trapped in the negative side of any positive/negative duality.

EITHER/OR THINKING, FOCUS, AND STRESS

When we focus on just one side of an Either/Or duality, and deny the existence of any other qualities, we significantly distort the truth about reality. And when we have a distorted view of reality, we can generate stress in our lives that would never have occurred if we had a broader and more accurate view of what actually happened.

Similarly, when we become aware that we have automatically become trapped within a very narrow, one-sided view of reality - for instance the negative side - and we then consciously choose to expand our focus to consider other legitimate viewpoints, we can prevent or eliminate much of the stress that did result, or would have resulted, from our previously distorted one-sided, negative perspectives.

Here again, we see the enormous influence of focus in our lives. Because we live (and grow up within) a society that conditions us to think in misleading Either/Or terms, our focus is restricted, in many cases, to just the negative side of a much broader reality.

On the other hand, we all have the ability to expand our focus...anytime we choose. Even though our bodies are programmed to think in Either/Or ways, we don't have to remain stuck in these narrow, one-sided perspectives. We can consciously choose to expand our view and consider other aspects of reality that may also be true at the very same time.

So the next time you automatically view something as being exclusively 'bad', or exclusively 'wrong' - consider testing out your awesome power to consciously redirect your focus. See if you can look from the opposite perspective and notice other 'truths' about reality that your initial, limited,   negative focus might have caused you to miss.

If you try this a few times, you might be surprised at what new things you will see. In fact, if you get very good at this handy refocusing skill, you might just find that some of your stress will magically disappear, even though your automatic negative thinking pattern hasn't changed one bit.

NOTE: Believe it or not, there are also many people who suffer from automatic positive thinking. This is just as much tied to Either/Or Thinking as negative thinking is - the only difference is that over time, automatic positive thinkers become conditioned to get trapped in just the positive view of any circumstance. As a result, they can't easily see or appreciate certain risks and potential dangers that may actually be present.

4

STOP BEING
A CONTROL FREAK

Here's an important tip that many negative thinkers never fully come to terms with. If you are a frequent negative thinker now, you've been a negative thinker for years. And if you've been a negative thinker for many years...this is not going to change for you. At least it's not going to change anytime in the near future. Possibly many years down the road it might, but certainly not now or anytime soon.

NEGATIVE THINKING IS A BODY PROBLEM...IT'S NOT A MENTAL PROBLEM

Most people incorrectly view negative thinking as a mental problem. By committing this fundamental mistake, they incorrectly assume that all it takes to 'fix' such a problem is to simply 'change your mind' or to simply 'control' your frequent negative thought processes.

But negative thinking is not really a mental problem at all. As we previously established, it is a body problem - it occurs because our bodies have been programmed (i.e. conditioned) to respond automatically with negative thoughts about all sorts of things that happen or that we are concerned might happen in the future.

Thus, the proper way to view negative thinking is to consider it a body problem. And this way of viewing negative thinking has important implications that many people fail to appreciate. These implications include:

> *You cannot easily 'change' or 'control' your negative thinking (if your body has been programmed over many years to habitually respond in negative thinking ways);*

> *Your negative thinking will continue to occur, even if you gain much more insight into it (from reading this guide, for example) than you ever had before;*

> *Over time, you may be able to recondition your body to think a bit more positively, but this can take many, many years to happen;*

> *There is no reason to blame yourself or criticize yourself for continuing to engage in*

automatic, negative thinking, once you become aware that your body has this tendency (it's just what your body's been programmed to do);

➤ *The best way to deal with negative thinking is not to fight it, try to stop it, try to control it, or otherwise resist it. The best way is to simply relax and just let it keep happening - as it will anyway - and then develop some new and better strategies for using your body's negative thinking tendencies to your advantage.*

STOP TRYING TO CONTROL YOUR NEGATIVE THINKING

Do yourself a favor right now and take a lot of pressure and frustration off yourself by giving up your pipedream that you'll eventually be able to stop or control your negative thinking. You won't be able to do this.

Even better, you don't need to stop or control your negative thinking in order to overcome it. This is a good thing, since trying to stop or control your negative thinking isn't likely to succeed, for the reasons cited above.

There are several things you can do, however, once you recognize that you (your body) has been programmed to automatically think in very negative ways. These things that you can do, and which I'll reveal later in this guide, can indeed allow you to overcome many of the stress-producing effects of your negative thinking - without having it change or go away at all.

5

HERE'S A PRESENT FOR YOU – ENJOY IT!

I now want to give you some pointers about how you can tell when your negative thinking is true and appropriate...and when it is not.

THERE ARE NO 'NEGATIVES' IN THE BOX CALLED 'LIFE'

You know how when you buy something from a store, and it comes in a big box, there's usually a list of all the contents inside of the box printed on the outside or on a separate sheet of paper located within the box. This list contains all the components that should be included in the box, and by inference, if something is not on the list, it's not in the box.

Well, in many ways this same analogy can be applied to life. There are certain things that come in the 'box' called 'life' and other things that don't. For example, in 'the box called life', you will find lots of living things and lots of non-living things.

In the category of living things, you will find plants, animals, bacteria, viruses, and human beings. You will find human bodies in the box. And you will find human language in the box. You will also find many events (or potential events) in the box.

But what you won't find in 'the box called life' is any negatives. Negatives are not part of life. Negatives only arise from human bodies and from human language. That's the only place they exist. They do not occur in life, per se.

MOST NEGATIVE THINKING IS FAULTY THINKING

If you understand this key principle that negatives don't come in the box called life, you should always be suspicious anytime you are thinking negatively. This is not to say that negative thinking doesn't have any value, or that it is always faulty or wrong. It's just to point out that the odds are very much in favor that most of our negative thoughts are going to be incomplete, incorrect, or otherwise unrealistic.

Thus, you should always treat your automatic, negative thinking as potentially flawed.

This should be your impetus for always trying to challenge and disprove any negative thoughts you might have. Sometimes, you won't be able to do this (meaning your negative thoughts may be just fine), but much of the time, you will be able to see through any weaknesses in your initial, automatic negative ideas.

POSITIVE THINKING CAN BE FLAWED AS WELL

As we've just seen, people who've gone through life and have bodies conditioned to think very positively tend to ignore risks, dangers, and other legitimate negative aspects of life. Thus, their automatic body tendencies can be just as flawed and just as inaccurate as our automatic negative thinking can be.

So it's not just negative thinking, or even positive thinking that is commonly flawed. All types of automatic, conditioned thinking are likely to be wrong much of the time.

This goes for automatic thought processes such as:

> ➤ *Our automatic assumptions.*
> ➤ *Our expectations about ourselves, about others, about life, etc.*
> ➤ *Our automatic ways of perceiving events in life.*
> ➤ *Our thoughts that automatically generate our emotions.*
> ➤ *Our theories that underlie our behaviors.*
> ➤ *Our judgments about other people.*

> ➢ *Our thoughts about our own value, worth, and lovability.*

> ➢ *Our thoughts about how to have successful relationships.*

And much, much more.

6

WHERE NEGATIVE THINKING REALLY COMES FROM

So, if there is no negativity in the box called life, where does negativity truly come from?

Well, if it doesn't come from life...it has to come from us! And in fact, it always does.

In a deeply philosophical (and truthful) way, nothing negative ever truly happens in life. There are no negative events in life, no negative situations, no negative outcomes, no negative people, no negative emotions, etc.

The truth is that things just keep on happening in life, and then we human beings either consciously or unconsciously add our interpretations to whatever happens. This is true for even the most severely 'negative' events we can imagine, such as natural disasters, genocide, senseless individual murders of innocent people, etc.

The truth of the matter is more like this:

> *Events happen in life and then we judge them to be either good or bad;*

> *Situations occur in each of our lives, and we assess them to be either positive or negative;*

> *Certain outcomes stem either directly or indirectly from our actions, and we then judge these outcomes to be favorable or unfavorable;*

> *Someone senselessly kills another person and we judge this to be bad or wrong.*

This is why it's so very important to know and continually remind yourself that nothing 'negative' ever happens in life.

Negativity is always a product of human interpretation. And sometimes, our automatic interpretations - particularly our automatic negative ones - can be way off the mark.

If you incorrectly assume that something you experience 'really is negative', then you will never consider exploring whether your own automatic assessments may not be correct.

This is also part of the root cause of our 'believing problem', which I mentioned in Point #1 of this plan. We tend to over-value and believe in our negative thoughts much more than we should. This is because we mistakenly believe they 'really are true' - as in they are true independent of us and   of our own or others' possibly faulty interpretations.

Once you recognize, however, that all negativity is a product of human interpretation, and none of it exists as a 'fact of nature', you are then freed up from your automatic negative thinking to explore other valid views of reality.

7

How's Your Relationship?

Have you ever heard the terms 'double whammy' or 'one-two punch' before? Sure you have. Well, if you are a negative thinker, you too have become the victim of a diabolical one-two double whammy.

Not only do you have a problem with automatic negative thinking - which is bad enough - but you also have a second problem as well. This problem is that you also have an automatic way of relating to your negative thinking whenever it occurs.

Even worse, while you may be consciously aware of your negative thoughts, when they occur, you may not be aware of your automatic way of relating to your negative thoughts, which is hidden much more deeply in the background. Thus, you haven't seen this second punch that is hitting you, so you haven't been able to defend yourself from it.

WHAT IS YOUR CURRENT RELATIONSHIP TO YOUR NEGATIVE THINKING?

I've already spilled the beans on this, earlier in this report, but you may not have connected the dots...yet. Your current relationship to your automatic negative thinking is to **automatically believe** that most of your negative thoughts are absolutely and unassailably true!

As I mentioned earlier, this is the heart of your negative thinking problem - not your negative thinking per se...which is what most people mistakenly believe is the underlying problem to be solved.

No. The underlying problem to be solved is how you automatically relate to your negative thinking - and this is the 'believing problem' I mentioned in Point #1.

Look, you can have hundreds of negative thoughts popping into your head all day long, and if you simply ignored or didn't pay any attention to 95% of them, you wouldn't suffer any major consequences from your negative thinking.

But that's not what you do. You not only DON'T IGNORE most of the negative thoughts that flow through your head every day, but you compound the problem by actually believing they are true, when the vast majority of them are not.

And what you may not be consciously aware of - until right now - is that you automatically assume your negative thoughts to be true, without subjecting them to any scrutiny or reality testing at all. If you did this, you would eventually find out how many of your automatic thoughts are distorted, incomplete, or just plain wrong. And after recognizing this a few thousand times, you'll eventually stop believing so strongly in them, and this will free you up to simply start ignoring them.

NOTE: There are several types of mindful meditation practices that can assist you in developing this skill. In these practices, you simply sit quietly in a comfortable position for 15-30 minutes or more and try not to move or respond to anything. You simply observe any thoughts, feelings, or body sensations that occur within your body, and then you practice the gentle but powerful art of just 'letting them be' or just letting them run through you for however long they last. You don't try to change them, control them, or even believe in them. You just simply observe them and whatever else occurs within your body. Even if you do have a random negative thought and notice that you are believing very strongly that it is true - just notice and observe that you are doing this and don't try to do anything about it. Just practice the ancient art of observing everything that automatically occurs within your body - for a short but defined period of time each day - and eventually, good things will start to happen for you.

THE ODDS ARE IN YOUR FAVOR - OR AGAINST YOU - DEPENDING ON HOW YOU LOOK AT IT

Remember what I told you earlier - most negative thinking is faulty thinking. This means that most of your negative thinking is likely to be incomplete, distorted, or even flat out wrong.

This also means the odds are way, way in your favor that if you start to critically examine each of your automatic negative thoughts from the perspective that each is in some way likely to be either partly or totally wrong, you will often find this to be the case. In particular, here are some additional types of negative thoughts that you should always seek to challenge, because the odds are extremely high (in some cases 100%) that your automatic assessments are not anywhere close to being true:

> ➤ *Negative thoughts about yourself and your future in life.*

> ➤ *Negative thoughts about other people's motives for doing the things they do.*

> ➤ *Negative thoughts about your ability to be happy and fulfilled in your life.*

> ➤ *Negative thoughts about whether you will ever find a suitable mate.*

> ➤ *Negative thoughts about problems you believe will never be solved or situations you believe could never be changed.*

> ➤ *Any thoughts you might have that you are stupid, weak, or a failure.*

> ➤ *Any thoughts you might have that you are unlovable.*

> ➤ *Any thoughts you might have that you are not as good or worthy as other people.*

> ➤ *Any regrets or recriminations you might have about anything you did (or didn't do) in the past.*

Etc.

8

CHANGING AUTOMATIC NEGATIVE ASSUMPTIONS

The interesting thing about how we habitually relate to anything in life is that, as human beings, we always have the power to change the way we are going to relate to something in the future - anytime we want.

In other words, we can choose to have a different relationship - different from our automatic, habitual one - and we don't need anyone else's permission or help to do so. We can simply decide to adopt a new relationship and presto - in the very next moment that new way of relating can be created and up and running for us. This really is quite magical.

If you don't believe me, all you have to do is recall or Google one of the most dramatic examples of this awesome power which emerged in the 1970s known as 'pet rocks'.

One day in the 1970s, someone in California got the bright marketing idea of accumulating a bunch of rocks, decorating them cleverly, and then selling them in bright packaging to lonely people who were encouraged to relate to them as their own personal pets. The benefits were a new source of friendship and comfort in your life, without all the fuss of having to feed, care for, walk, or clean up after a real pet, which after all can be demanding.

This marketing concept caught on briefly and spread like wildfire. In a very short time, thousands of people had purchased and were giddy about their new 'pet rocks'.

In retrospect, this phenomenon was not all that astonishing. Again, as human beings we have the ability to change our relationships to anything - even a dull rock. One day, a rock can just be a rock to you. The next day, it can be your best friend whom you will protect and defend 'till your death.

The key thing to notice here is that nothing about the rock had to change. Instead of buying a high-priced, decorated rock (plus fashion accessories), you could have just gone out in your back yard and found a new pet rock for free (as many people eventually did). The only thing that had to change was your relationship to that rock, and this is entirely within your own personal power to determine.

In the very same way, when you set out to change your relationship to the negative thoughts that constantly run through your head, nothing at all needs to change about them. They can happen just as often as they did before, they can be just as negative, and they can be just as faulty as before - nothing about them needs to change.

The only thing that needs to change is your relationship to them. What this means is:

> *Instead of automatically resisting them and wishing they would stop bothering you, you voluntarily choose to do something else.*

> *Instead of hating them and viewing them as something destructive in your life, you create a new relationship to them that has them be of benefit to you.*

> *Instead of automatically assuming that each of your negative thoughts is necessarily true, you create a new relationship where you begin to examine and question each and every one of them.*

PRACTICE COMBATING YOUR AUTOMATIC NEGATIVE ASSUMPTIONS

Once again, you already have an automatic, habitual relationship to your negative thoughts, and this relationship can be summed up by saying that you automatically and sincerely believe them to be true.

> ### You have got to start changing this relationship ... and you've got to start this today!

You've got to stop believing that every silly, negative thought that enters your head is valid. Most of them are not. Even the very serious ones. But you've so practiced and perfected the habit of believing them to be true that you're reluctant to do the hard work of constantly reminding yourself that they're probably not.

The automatic negative thoughts you have are *lying to you* most of the time.

So instead of continuing to practice believing they are true, you need to start practicing the opposite skill - challenging them and reminding yourself that your assumptions of negativity are way overblown.

DON'T RESIST YOUR NEGATIVE THINKING

Remember, your automatic negative thinking is best viewed as a body problem - not a mental problem. It continually occurs because our bodies have been programmed (i.e. conditioned) to automatically respond with negative thought patterns when we are triggered in certain ways.

I also suggested earlier in this guide that:

> *"The best way to deal with negative thinking is not to fight it, try to stop it, try to control it, or otherwise resist it.*
>
> *The best way is to simply relax and just let it keep happening - as it will do anyway - and then develop some new strategies for how to best use your body's negative thinking tendencies to your advantage."*

So just accept the fact that you (actually your body) is going to continue to think negatively, and there's little you can do to stop this.

Fortunately, there's no need to resist your negative thinking. You can relax and just let it keep happening. The key is to have a few strategies in place (i.e. adopt a new relationship) to deal with your negative thinking whenever it automatically occurs.

IT ALL STARTS WITH SELF-AWARENESS

The key to adopting new strategies for dealing with negative thinking is becoming more aware of when your body has been triggered to think negatively.

Believe it or not, many negative thinkers are not consciously aware that their bodies have been triggered to think negatively. They just go through life, having multiple negative thoughts and perceptions every day, thinking that this is just the way life really is, and it has little to do with them, their automatic interpretations, or their bodies.

On the other hand, once you become aware that your body has been programmed to think negatively, a whole new world of choices suddenly opens up for you. For example, once you notice that you are having negative thoughts, you could ask yourself the following new types of questions:

> **?** *"Isn't it interesting that my body tends to focus on negatives in these specific situations?"*

> **?** *"Is it true that whatever just happened really was negative?"*

> **?** *"Are there any positive aspects to whatever happened that I might be missing?"*

? *"Even if what did happen appears to be negative, is there any way I could turn it into something positive?"*

USE YOUR NEGATIVE THINKING AS A PERSONAL WAKE-UP CALL

You could even adopt a strategy where you utilize your body's tendency to frequently think negatively as an internal 'wake-up call'. Here's how this creative strategy might work:

1. Let yourself think negatively whenever your body wants;

2. Improve your ability to recognize (i.e. become consciously aware of) when you have been triggered to think negatively;

3. Decide that whenever you notice yourself thinking negatively, you will use this as a **warning signal** to begin looking for positive aspects that your automatic negative thinking may have caused you to miss.

Once again, the beauty of this type of strategy and new relationship to your automatic thinking is that it doesn't require you to stop, change, or control your negative thinking at all. You don't have to fight or resist your body's automatic tendencies. You can simply relax, go 'with the flow', and just have a few simple strategies on hand to keep your negative thinking from getting you into trouble, or from causing you needless stress and suffering.

9

Would You Rather Be Right or Happy?

Here's a trick question for you: if you are a frequent negative thinker, how often do you suppose you are wrong?

I say this is a trick question because I've already answered it.

You are going to be wrong much more often than you think. In fact, you can take whatever percentage you came up with, say 5-10% of the time - and multiply that number by 10!

Remember, Socrates was able to show the best and brightest thinkers in Ancient Greece that most of what they believed to be true was deeply wrong, and these weren't even all negative thinkers. So why do you think you are any smarter?

Actually, we are all frequently wrong much of the time in life, whether we are positive, negative, or completely balanced thinkers. This is just part of being human, and there's little we can do to avoid it.

But if you're a frequent negative thinker, this means you're going to be wrong a much higher percentage of the time than people who are not negative thinkers—for the reasons outlined earlier in this guide.

Therefore, it pays to always be very suspicious of each and every negative thought you might have. And don't forget, every time you have a negative feeling, such as anger, guilt, fear, worry, sadness, etc., guess what? Negative thoughts are lurking in the background to produce these negative feelings. So don't automatically assume that your negative feelings, as attached as you may be to them, are necessarily true as well.

> *The good news is that if you create the right relationship to your automatic negative thinking, you actually can become much wiser and more accurate in your thinking than ever before.*

If you take my advice and use your negative thinking as a personal wake up call to motivate you to search for alternate, positive views of reality, your scope of awareness will be expanded and you'll be able to see more of the truth about what's really going on around you.

10

FLIP TO THE OPPOSITE REALITY

The 'secret sauce' for overcoming negative thinking is not to try to stop your negative thoughts or change them in any way. It's not even to force yourself to think more positively. Rather, it's to allow your negative thoughts to keep occurring, as often as they want, and then know how to defeat them and keep them from causing mischief in your life - by learning how to challenge and successfully disprove them.

WHY POSITIVE THINKING DOESN'T WORK

I am now able to explain to you why positive thinking doesn't work and why, despite its popularity, it is a very flawed strategy for dealing with negative thinking.

WHAT IS POSITIVE THINKING?

Positive Thinking is a strategy that is widely promoted for dealing with negative thinking. When you use this strategy, you try to overpower your body's tendency to think negatively by forcing yourself to think more positive thoughts.

The theory behind this strategy is that you can overpower negative thinking with the sheer force of your mental willpower and thereby cause yourself to think more positively.

WHAT'S WRONG WITH POSITIVE THINKING?

This strategy is flawed for several reasons. First, it causes you to fight against, resist, and try to overpower your body's tendency to think in a negative fashion. This is very hard work and requires a great deal of forceful psychological effort.

The second drawback is that this strategy assumes you can 'push' your negative thinking out of existence (i.e. make it go away) by replacing it with more forceful positive thoughts. Actually, your negative thinking doesn't go away at all. It's still there, deep within your body. All you manage to do with Positive Thinking is hide it from your view.

The Influence Of 'Internal Realities'

The main problem with Positive Thinking is that it fails to take into account certain features of the human body. One of the most important of these features is the way our automatic, conditioned ways of thinking produce 'internal realities' (i.e. conclusions, perceptions, feelings, etc.) that our bodies then automatically 'assume to be true'.

Our bodies react emotionally and physiologically to these 'assumed to be true internal realities' - not to the reality of whatever may have happened outside of us.

When you try to use Positive Thinking to overpower your body's automatic tendency to think negatively - and to assume your negative thinking is absolutely true - you do nothing to release the hold your 'internal realities' have on your body. You just give yourself the false impression that they have actually been dealt with and have therefore gone away.

But they're still there - having effects upon your body - whether you're aware of this or not.

In other words, Positive Thinking does nothing to address the 'believing problem' which is the deeper and more important problem to solve. When you deeply believe that your initial automatic thoughts really are true, no amount of positive counter-thinking, or positive affirmations, is going to hold any credible sway with you. Deep down inside, you are still going to believe that your negative thoughts and assumptions really are true.

CHALLENGING AND DISPROVING NEGATIVE THOUGHTS

Instead of using Positive Thinking, you should try to challenge and disprove (or see beyond) your automatic negative thoughts instead. This is very different from trying to suppress, avoid, or overpower them with more positive thoughts. You simply let your negative thoughts occur, bring them out into the open (as opposed to trying to suppress or overpower them), and then you *critically examine them* and ask yourself if they are really true and appropriate to your situation at hand.

Often, when you do this, you will find that a more positive perspective emerges - but not because you forced yourself to adopt it (while your body was still holding on to an exclusively negative belief). What causes a more positive perspective to naturally emerge is that you successfully examined and 'destroyed' a false negative 'internal reality' that your body had been endorsing very strongly.

For example, if you are feeling angry (about anything), you can be sure that certain 'internal realities' became triggered within your body to produce your emotion of anger. Now, you can try to force yourself to believe you are not angry (even though you are) through Positive Thinking, if you want.

But your body will still be holding on to the assumed-to-be true **negative internal realities** that are driving your anger in the first place. So from you body's standpoint, you would still be angry (and this can be documented physiologically) no matter how many positive thoughts you forced yourself to think.

On the other hand, when you bring your anger-producing internal realities out into the open (instead of forcing them deep into the background), and when you successfully challenge and disprove them, you anger will lessen because you will have 'destroyed' the internal driving forces that brought it about and that are responsible for maintaining it.

I hope you can see that this is both a very different process, and a very different outcome, from what happens with Positive Thinking.

WHAT IS 'FLIPPING TO THE OPPOSITE REALITY'?

When you start out trying to challenge and disprove your frequent negative thoughts, this can be a bit difficult at first. Mostly, this is because you probably haven't practiced this skill very much in the past.

Secondly, you can often draw a blank when it comes to considering other not-so-negative viewpoints, which may not come easily to mind.

One handy technique for zeroing in on your negative thoughts and discovering alternative (valid) viewpoints is to take any single negative thought and turn it completely on its head. Simply take that thought and turn it around to its total opposite - then **look from that opposite perspective** and see what you can see.

Notice that I didn't say take that opposite perspective and believe it. I'm not asking you to force yourself to accept or believe anything. All I'm suggesting is that you can use this artificial conceptual device to focus your attention in a specific opposite direction that is not usually automatic for you.

Once you consider this opposite perspective, you will either see things about your present situation that you can honestly admit are also true - or you won't. So you only have to accept and believe in whatever truly occurs to you to believe.

Example: You think someone did something really bad and wrong, and you are really struggling to relinquish your automatic belief in this assessment and to look at what happened in any other way. Try 'Flipping To The Opposite Reality' and think of it like a humorous party game. Try asking yourself :"Is there any way what this person did might actually have been good or might have been right for them to do?"

Just take this opposite reality view and see what you see when you think from this totally made up vantage point.

You may just be surprised to find that you really can see ways that this opposite may be true as well (in contrast to your automatic negative assumptions).

Try this out a few times, and I think you'll be pretty amazed at how often it works! And remember, for the reasons mentioned above, that this has nothing to do with positive thinking, even though you might end up naturally thinking much more positive thoughts.

NOTE: I have an entire chapter-length appendix on how to use this technique, and why it works so well, in my award-winning book The 14 Day Stress Cure, which you can learn more about at:

http://14daystresscure.com

CONCLUSION

By purchasing and reading this guide, you now have a ten-point success plan to follow for reducing any adverse effects that negative thinking might otherwise have in your life.

Here is a recap of the ten key points in your plan:

1. Negative thinking isn't your real problem...believing your negative thinking is!

2. Your body has become conditioned to automatically focus on negatives, thereby making you blind to other valid aspects of reality.

3. Either/Or Thinking repeatedly gets you into trouble because it sets you up to focus mainly on negatives and discount positives.

4. You can't stop thinking negatively, even if you want to, so you need to let go of this unrealistic pipedream.

5. Nothing negative ever happens in life.

6. Any negatives that appear to be part of life actually come from our internal thoughts, interpretations, and assessments.

7. Your present relationship to your negative thinking is to automatically assume that it is true.

8. The best relationship to have towards your negative thinking is to assume just the opposite - that much of your negative thinking is wrong or highly distorted.

9. If you are human, you're going to be wrong a good bit of the time. If you are a negative thinker, you are going to be wrong even more, because negative thinking is frequently faulty thinking.

10. One trick to help you challenge and disprove your automatic negative thoughts is to 'flip to the opposite reality' and see what you can validate when you look from this perspective.

Good luck with your efforts to stop having your life be dominated by negative thinking. If this guide does help you accomplish this goal, please let me know by emailing me your success story at:

docorman@gmail.com

To your health, happiness, and success,

Doc Orman, M.D.

P.S. If you liked this book, I am developing an international community of like-minded people who are interested in achieving higher levels of stress reduction than stress management can provide.

I am building this community through my Stress Mastery Academy, and you are welcome to join us if you'd like. The cost is a one-time fee of less than $10, and this includes an excellent advanced training course on how to master stress, along with a subscription to our 52-week email newsletter.

You can find out more about how to join this Academy by going to www.stressmasteryacademy.com and downloading the free special report featured there.

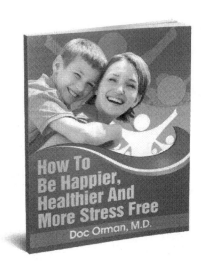

At the end of this report, you'll learn all about the Academy and the advanced training course you'll receive when you join.

OTHER BOOKS BY DOC ORMAN

Stress Relief Wisdom: Ten Key Distinctions For A Stress Free Life

The Choice Of Paradox: How "Opposite Thinking" Can Improve Your Life And Reduce Your Stress

The Ultimate Method For Dealing With Stress: How To Eliminate Anxiety, Irritability And Other Types Of Stress Without Having To Use Drugs, Relaxation Exercises Or Stress Management Techniques

The Art Of True Forgiveness: How To Forgive Anyone For Anything, Anytime You Want

The Irritability Cure: How To Stop Being Angry, Anxious and Frustrated All The Time

The Test Anxiety Cure: How To Overcome Exam Anxiety, Fear and Self Defeating Habits

The 14 Day Stress Cure: A New Approach For Dealing With Stress That Can Change Your Life

How To Have A Stress Free Wedding...And Live
Happily Ever After

Sleep Well Again: How To Fall Asleep Fast, Stay
Asleep Longer, And Get Better Sleep Like You
Did In The Past

About The Author

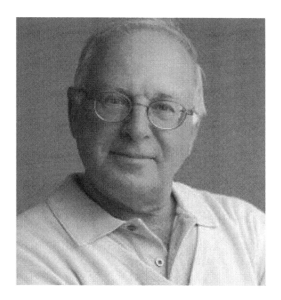

MORT (Doc) ORMAN, M.D. is an Internal Medicine physician, author, stress coach, and founder of the Stress Mastery Academy. He has been teaching people how to eliminate stress, without managing it, for more than 30 years. He has also conducted seminars and workshops on reducing stress for doctors, nurses, veterinarians, business executives, students, the clergy, and even the F.B.I.

Dr. Orman's award-winning book, The 14 Day Stress Cure (1991), is still one of the most helpful and innovative books on the subject of stress ever written. Dr. Orman and his wife, Christina, a veterinarian, live in Maryland.

77484270R00042

Made in the USA
Middletown, DE
21 June 2018